OTHER BOOKS BY ALEX MITCHELL

Quizzin' Nine-Nine: A *Brooklyn Nine-Nine* Quiz Book

Parks & Interrogation: A *Parks & Recreation* Quiz Book

Q & AC-12: A *Line of Duty* Quiz Book

Know Your Schitt: A *Schitt's Creek* Quiz Book

Examilton: A *Hamilton* Quiz Book

Stranger Thinks: A *Stranger Things* Quiz Book

The El Clued Brothers: A *Peep Show* Quiz Book

Dunder Quizlin: An *Office US* Quiz Book

A Question of Succession: A *Succession* Quiz Book

The Big Bang Queries: A *Big Bang Theory* Quiz Book

The Greendale Study Guide: A *Community* Quiz Book

Peaky Masterminders: A *Peaky Blinders* Quiz Book

The First-Time Parent's Quiz Book

A Quiz Per Week to Guide Parents-To-Be Through Pregnancy & Beyond

Alex Mitchell

Published by Beartown Press

Copyright © 2021 Alex Mitchell

ISBN: 9798711198949

The moral right of the author has been asserted. All rights reserved. No part of this publication may be reproduced, stored in a retrieval system, or transmitted in any form or by any means, without the prior permission in writing from the publisher.

Please note that the author is not a doctor, and that the answers provided within these pages do not replace medical advice from your healthcare provider. Information around pregnancy and newborns continually changes; the contents of this book are based on information available at the time of writing.

1st Edition.

Contents

Introduction	7
The First Trimester	9
Weeks One & Two	11
Week Three	13
Week Four	15
Week Five	17
Week Six	20
Week Seven	22
Week Eight	24
Week Nine	26
Week Ten	28
Week Eleven	31
Week Twelve	33
Week Thirteen	35
The Second Trimester	**37**
Week Fourteen	39
Week Fifteen	41
Week Sixteen	43
Week Seventeen	46
Week Eighteen	49
Week Nineteen	51
Week Twenty	53
Week Twenty-One	56
Week Twenty-Two	58

Week Twenty-Three	60
Week Twenty-Four	62
Week Twenty-Five	65
Week Twenty-Six	67
Week Twenty-Seven	70
The Third Trimester	**73**
Week Twenty-Eight	75
Week Twenty-Nine	78
Week Thirty	81
Week Thirty-One	83
Week Thirty-Two	85
Week Thirty-Three	87
Week Thirty-Four	89
Week Thirty-Five	91
Week Thirty-Six	94
Week Thirty-Seven	97
Week Thirty-Eight	100
Week Thirty-Nine	102
Week Forty	104
Weeks Forty-One & Forty-Two	106

Introduction

Hi, thanks for picking up this book, the majority of which I wrote over the course of my wife's pregnancy with our first child.

I'm definitely not comparing my own Herculean efforts in creating a quiz book to those of my wife in creating a human, by the way, although I do enjoy her reaction when I tell her it was a productive nine months for us both. (I'm always careful to do this from a distance.)

Mostly I thought this would be a good thing to do because - like every parent ever - I discovered there's a lot to learn during the baffling time in which you're expecting and then suddenly looking after your first baby, and my stupid brain can often only take stuff in if it's part of a game or something competitive. I thought a week-by-week quiz might be a nice, fun way to package some of the information.

In reality, of course, neither pregnancy nor parenting are a test that you, me or anyone else will ever score 100% in. The exam paper changes every day, bringing new questions that you've never even considered before, and the right answers for one person might not be the right ones for you.

And even the right answers for you today might not be the right answers for you tomorrow. There are no right answers, really.

It sounds like a moral from the end of a *Captain Planet* episode, but all you can really do as a parent is your best. You and I will both learn from our mistakes, borrow advice from a hundred different sources and ultimately make things up as we go along to create our own rules for ourselves and our babies. And it'll all work out in the end, because we care. You wouldn't be reading this if you didn't.

One last thing: I'm from the UK and my baby knowledge has all been gathered in a specific period of time. I've done my best to make the questions universal and futureproof, but guidance changes over time and will vary from country to country, so please always do check with your practitioner.

Good luck with your baby journey, and I hope you enjoy the book.

Have a great baby.

Alex.

The First Trimester

In which you discover a lot of things - from bewildering medical facts that might freak you out a little at first, to your own reaction to the fact you're expecting a real-life, human baby.

It's the time to dream and talk about how you might raise your child, what you might name them and how you might tell your families.

Trimester one also ushers in a significant gear change in general daily comfort levels if you're the one physically carrying the baby - all I can recommend is to use the support you have around you where you can.

That might mean tapping up parent friends for ideas to relieve some of the discomfort (my wife's first trimester was sponsored by her pregnancy pillow and Gaviscon), switching up things at home, such as which items are routinely bought in the big shop and who looks after particular household tasks, or arranging to work from home if your job allows it.

Pregnancy is a rollercoaster, to paraphrase Ronan Keating. You just have to ride it.

Weeks One & Two

Current baby size: Doesn't exist yet
Congratulations, you're expecting a baby! Although, weirdly, for the first two weeks of 'pregnancy', your baby is yet to be conceived (go figure), so this is more of a pre-emptive congrats...

This week's quiz
1. Which date is the starting point used to calculate a mother's due date, so is treated as the first day of the pregnancy?

2. How soon after ovulation is the egg fertilised?

3. What percentage chance does the average healthy couple have of conceiving in a given month, when trying?

4. How many trimesters are in a pregnancy?

5. Forget the classic Hollywood instant-morning-sickness scene. What's typically the first reliable sign of pregnancy?

A fun activity for this week

If you've not yet conceived, it's a good idea to make the most of doing things you won't really be able to do for the next nine months: go on an adventurous holiday, eat sushi, take part in a marathon and so on. It could be a long time until you're able to do them again!

Baby name inspiration

Game of Thrones. Think Arya, Tyrion, Daenerys, Ramsay, Jamie, Sansa and The Mountain. (Though I prefer 'The Mountain' as a middle name.)

Quiz answers

1. The first day of the mother's last period. Craziness, but who am I to challenge the system?
2. Within 24 hours - although sperm can live in the body for up to 5 or 6 days, so it can be useful to try having sex well before ovulation if you're trying for a baby.
3. About 20-25%.
4. Three, each lasting about thirteen weeks.
5. A missed period. Symptom spotting is not very helpful, in my experience. Best to wait for cast-iron indicators that something has changed.

Week Three

Current baby size: Vanilla bean seed

OK, great news: now you're actually pregnant! You probably don't know it yet, but a sperm and an egg have been introduced, they've got on like a house on fire, and now, somewhere in a uterus near you, there's a tight little bunch of fast-multiplying cells that will eventually become your baby.

This week's quiz

1. A pregnancy test checks for the presence of which hormone in a woman's body in order to deliver a positive result?

2. How many cells is the fertilised egg (also known as a zygote) that will become your baby made up of to begin with?

3. True or false: Home pregnancy tests are always accurate?

4. Nutrition is very important during pregnancy. How many extra calories should a woman be eating during her first trimester?

5. Into which organ does the embryo implant?

A fun activity for this week

Make your list for the weekly big shop and factor in the various things that your pregnant self or pregnant are going to need to switch from and to. Out with the regular coffee beans and alcohol, in with the decaf and the mocktails.

Baby name inspiration

The Kardashians. I'm thinking Kim, Kourtney, Kris, Kendall, Kylie, Khloe, Kraig and Kolin. And, by extension, Kanye.

Quiz answers

1. HCG (or human chorionic gonadotropin). This hormone is created in a woman's placenta after a fertilized egg implants in her uterus.
2. One. But it quickly divides into much more than that - it's made up of over 100 calls within just a few days. Amazing.
3. False. A positive result is almost certainly correct, but a negative test result can be less reliable - especially if you're taking the test early or you're on particular medication.
4. None. According to the UK's National Institute for Health and Clinical Excellence (NICE): "Energy needs do not change in the first six months of pregnancy. Only in the last three months do a woman's energy needs increase by around 200 calories per day." Eat well, and eat healthily, but it seems there's no need to "eat for two"!
5. The uterus, AKA baby's home for the next nine months.

Week Four

Current baby size: Poppy seed

There's a good chance you'll find out that you're expecting either this week or quite soon afterwards - how exciting!

This week's quiz

1. While pregnant, it's best to avoid hair colouring until at least what stage of the pregnancy?

2. Around now, the cells of the newly-developing placenta begin producing human chorionic gonadotropin, or hCG, to nurture the fertilised egg. What is the side effect of hCG?

3. What is the average weight gain during pregnancy for women with a normal BMI?

4. What is a mum-to-be's recommended daily maximum intake of caffeine during her pregnancy?

5. At this stage you'll be looking forward to your dating scan to give you an idea of when to expect your little arrival - but how far into the pregnancy does it normally take place?

A fun activity for this week

Come up with the name by which you and your partner are going to refer to your little pup while they're hanging out in the bump for the next eight-or-so months. Common ones include Peanut, Spud, Jellybean and Bambi, but people come up with all sorts of weird and wonderful ones!

Baby name inspiration

Place of conception. Depending on what sounds best, this might be country (e.g. India, Chad), city (e.g. London, Brooklyn), borough (Kensington, Charlton) or even hotel (Belgravia, Travelodge).

Quiz answers

1. Until the second trimester at the very earliest. Research is limited, and the chemicals in hair dyes aren't hugely toxic, but it's generally considered safest to wait until after your first 12 weeks when the risk to your baby is much lower.
2. Morning sickness, or just general nausea. Yay, nature!
3. 11-14 kgs, or 25-32 lbs.
4. 200mg at time of writing - though always check with your practitioner.
5. 12 weeks in the UK, or around 6 to 9 weeks in the USA.

Week Five

Current baby size: Apple seed

This week your baby is looking decidedly tadpole-ish - he's pretty much a head and a tail at this stage. But don't worry, he's changing quickly and well on his way to being a fully-qualified baby. It's even possible that an ultrasound can pick up his little heartbeat this week (although this is more common in weeks 6 or 7). Cute.

This week's quiz

1. Different cultures have different beliefs about baby development. What hair-related tradition do Hindu fathers sometimes take part in?

2. Is a woman more likely to produce twins naturally if she's under 35 or if she's over 35?

3. Of your baby's different biological systems (cast your mind back to high school science class), which is the first to become operational?

4. Your baby's neural tube is also forming fast around now. Where does this run from and to inside his body?

5. Your HcG levels will be high enough at this stage to create a positive pregnancy test. You might want to shout the news from the rooftops, but when do people typically wait to tell friends and colleagues?

A fun activity for this week
You're not that far away from the mind-altering experience of parenthood, so you don't have long left with the perspective on things that you have today. With that in mind, try writing your future baby the occasional letter - give them advice, talk about what else is going on in your life, tell them stories about your past. I did this for a decent chunk of my wife's pregnancy and I don't know exactly when I intend to show the letters to my son (the content ranges from what we watched on TV last night to future career advice), but I suspect they're going to be interesting to look back on.

Baby name inspiration
Club legends from your favourite football team. In my case this is Port Vale, so unfortunately it doesn't get much more exotic than John, Neil, Gareth, Roy, Robin and Thomas.

Quiz answers
1. They part the hair on their pregnant partner's head three times, from front to back.

2. Over. Women over 35 produce lots of follicle-stimulating hormones and more follicles, both of which increase the chance of her releasing two or more eggs during ovulation.

3. Their adorable little circulatory system, as their heart begins pumping blood around their little body.

4. From his head to his rump - it'll go on to become his spinal cord.

5. Until after the third month, when many of the risks to your baby greatly reduce. It is totally up to you though and it's now much more common to tell people earlier than this.

Week Six

Current baby size: Sweet pea

This week your baby is busy diligently forming their lungs, kidneys and liver. Those lungs will be getting plenty of use when they're finally outside of the uterus - enjoy the peace and quiet while you can!

This week's quiz

1. Your baby will have measured a diminutive 4mm from crown to rump last week. What do they measure this week?

2. Pytalism is a typical side effect of pregnancy. But what does it actually mean?

3. How many weeks does a full-term pregnancy last?

4. You might be thinking about getting away for a break before the bubba arrives. What the latest week of pregnancy in which you're allowed to fly?

5. What is the first organ to actually form in your baby?

A fun activity for this week

Thinking about how you'll keep the pregnancy a secret from friends and family for a little while longer, if you have any social events approaching. Some friends of mine once spent an entire wedding reception swapping two identical glasses of wine back and forth between them, so that the wine was disappearing but the father-to-be was the only one drinking it. Unfortunately the side-effect of this was that the father-to-be ended up incredibly drunk and accidentally told several people throughout the day anyway.

Baby name inspiration

Disney characters. Elsa, Anna, Belle, Minnie, Jasmine, Flynn, Eric, Sven, Buzz, Milo and Cogsworth.

Quiz answers

1. 8mm. They've doubled in size in one week, a little like me over Christmas.
2. Excess saliva. So that's something to look forward to. Fortunately it usually subsides in later pregnancy!
3. 40 weeks. (It's considered around 38 weeks if you're carrying twins.)
4. Week 37, though some airlines and situations will prevent you from flying earlier.
5. The heart. Your baby has a lot of growing to do, so it's crucial that all of their cells can get the nutrients they need.

Week Seven

Current baby size: Blueberry
This week your baby's brain is manufacturing around a hundred new nerve cells every minute as their little nervous system begins to form. Remember, one day in the not-too-distant future they'll be showing you how to set up a technical new home device of some kind.

This week's quiz
1. In 1965 in the UK, just 5% of dads attended the birth of their children. What percentage of dads attend the birth as of 2020?

2. During her pregnancy, the average woman's breasts grow by how much (in both cms and lbs)?

3. The CDC and NHS suggest taking a folic acid supplement while you're trying to get pregnant, as well as for the first 12 weeks of your pregnancy, in order to reduce the chance of certain birth defects. But what daily dosage do they recommend?

4. Which exercise helps to prepare a woman's body for the pushing required during labour?

5. You might be experiencing some nausea already at this stage in your pregnancy - sorry about that! - but you're not alone. What percentage of mothers-to-be suffer from nausea at some point during their pregnancy?

A fun activity for this week
Work out an exercise routine that can evolve through the rest of your pregnancy. It might be as simple as adding a yoga session or a long weekend walk into your routine, and there's plenty of watch-along YouTube sessions to get involved in.

Baby name inspiration
Celebrity baby names. There's plenty to go at here. Apple, Jermajesty, Rumer, Scout, Moon Unit, Dweezil, Billion, North, Birdie and, of course, little X Æ A-Xii.

Quiz answers
1. 96%.
2. 5cm and 3lbs each. It's best to set aside decent budget for comfortable nursing bras that can also be worn through pregnancy.
3. 400 micrograms per day, at time of writing – though, of course, always check with your practitioner.
4. Pelvic floor exercises. And great news - there's no reason partners can't join in and it's never too early to start!
5. 70-80%.

Week Eight

Current baby size: Raspberry

At the end of eight weeks, you're officially 20% of the way through your pregnancy (and this book)! While that first chunk probably seems to have passed quite quickly, in my experience the next 15 weeks will pass quite slowly as you wait for the scans and checkups that get you a little bit closer to your cub. It's a good time to get into that lengthy TV series that you can binge-watch.

This week's quiz

1. Approximately how fast is your baby's heart beating at this stage?

2. What is the name of the liquid that forms in the womb to help cushion a baby throughout pregnancy?

3. Which of the following activities can cause babies to be born smaller than expected: smoking, drinking or intense exercising?

4. What is Couvade syndrome, which can occur during a pregnancy?

5. What proportion of women experience symptoms of depression during pregnancy?

A fun activity for this week
Start watching documentaries about first-time parents coping with their newborns. BBC's *The Baby Has Landed* was one we got into. I will point out here that we found documentaries about actual labour and the delivery process too stressful. The good thing is that you discover a lot of possibilities you weren't aware of. The bad thing is that you discover a lot of possibilities you weren't aware of.

Baby name inspiration
Jazz legends. I'm talking Louis, Duke, Miles, Billie, Buddy, Ella, Thelonius, Nina, Woody and so on. Your little one could be the coolest kid in the playground.

Quiz answers
1. Around 160 beats per minute.
2. Amniotic fluid.
3. Smoking.
4. It's where an expectant father experiences symptoms like morning sickness, backache, mood swings and food cravings. It's thought it can happen when a man is so deeply involved in a pregnancy.
5. One in ten. So be mindful of this, and be kind to yourself/your partner - especially during the down times.

Week Nine

Current baby size: Green olive

The first trimester of pregnancy can be tough, and it's around now that the toughness really ramps up. Nausea. Tiredness. Moodswings. Greasy skin. It's not dissimilar to being a teenager after a night out, actually. Except that this time it's 24/7 and bundled up with all of the anxieties that come with the countdown to becoming a parent.

But don't worry, there's light at the end of the tunnel: the second trimester is on its way, and that one's much more enjoyable.

This week's quiz

1. By how many times its original size does a woman's uterus grow during pregnancy?

2. During pregnancy, is a woman's voice more likely to get higher, or deeper?

3. What decides your baby's gender - the egg or the sperm?

4. Which one of the following CAN you eat during pregnancy: sushi, goat's cheese, liver or hard-boiled eggs?

5. How often is a new baby born globally?

A fun activity for this week
Find a social drink you can enjoy to replace the wine, beer or spirits of pre-pregnancy. With a lot of things being off-limits during pregnancy, it's nice to still be able to share a bottle of something that's not also aimed at children. Mocktails and non-alcoholic wines are decent options, but personally I'd recommend non-alcoholic gin, which often tastes a lot like the real thing and can be kept interesting by stocking up on different tonics and other mixers.

Baby name inspiration
The fastest people in the world. Usain, Florence, Tyson, Tori, Carmelita, Justin, Donovan, Marion and Frankie.

Quiz answers
1. Up to 500 times!
2. Deeper. Increased oestrogen and progesterone levels can cause vocal swelling, making it harder to hit higher notes and easier to hit lower ones. Could be a good time to join a choir...
3. The sperm. The egg will always carry an X chromosome. Each sperm will carry either an X (for a girl) or a Y (for a boy).
4. Hard-boiled eggs - but the yolk has to be solid.
5. Every three seconds. There was at least one born during the time it took you to read this answer!

Week Ten

Current baby size: Lime

Your baby's face is really coming along now. Their head is too big for their little body at the moment, but they already have eyes, eyelids, a mouth and taste buds. They even have a tiny nose with two little nostrils. And in just seven short months you'll be face-to-face with that face, falling in love with the unique mix of you and your partner's genes and features.

This week's quiz

1. What is the best position to sleep in while pregnant?

2. Pregnant women often find that which of their senses heightens during their pregnancy?

3. How many sets of quadruplets are born in the US each year?

4. What is the longest an embryo has reportedly been frozen for before successfully producing a baby?

5. True or false: it is safe to exercise while pregnant?

A fun activity for this week

Take plenty of photos of your pregnancy journey. It might feel right now like it's never going to end, but it'll seem like a lifetime ago once your baby is here. Whether it's weekly 'bumpies' of the burgeoning belly or general shots of nursery assembly and other DIY, it's great to look back on.

Baby name inspiration

Greek mythology is brimming with interesting names. You've got the likes of Atlas, Castor, Jason, Orion, Pollux, Troy and Zeus for boys, and Asteria, Aura, Clio, Echo, Iris, Maia, Pandora and Rhea.

Quiz answers

1. On one's side, and ideally the left side for circulation purposes. Experts say that this avoids resting the weight of a quickly-growing uterus on veins, back, intestines and other important stuff during the second and third trimesters.
2. Their sense of smell. This is unfortunately a contributory factor in morning sickness and the sudden dislike of foods that were previously enjoyed.
3. Around 500. Having consulted a calculator I can confirm that's 2000 babies in total.
4. 12 years. It was for a pair of twins, born in Jerusalem in 2003. I feel like this could be the jumping-off point for some kind of time-travel thriller.

5. True AND false. In theory, exercising and staying healthy will help give you an easier pregnancy and more stamina for when you're in labour. However, it's best to avoid certain activities (walking and swimming can be great; high-impact activities like running less so) and some women have conditions such as preeclampsia that will prevent them from being able to safely exercise during pregnancy. Talk to your practitioner to understand what's best for your specific circumstances and stage of pregnancy.

Week Eleven

Current baby size: Prune

One quarter down, just three more to go. If you could see your baby right about now, you might be able to attempt a pinky shake to introduce yourselves. That's because your baby's fingers and toes are starting to separate on their previously-webbed hands and feet. And the cutest thing? They're starting to grow little fingernails and toenails. Aw.

This week's quiz

1. Around this time you'll know how many babies you're carrying - but what is the highest amount of babies delivered in a single pregnancy?

2. What actually *is* the placenta?

3. True or false: while they're still in the womb, babies can taste what their mother is eating?

4. Your baby will be urinating in the womb before long, if they're not already, and they'll pee up to a litre every day. But where does the urine disappear to?

5. True or false: babies are born with kneecaps?

A fun activity for this week

Stock up on your favourite complex carbs and proteins to help keep your blood sugar levels up through pregnancy. Try bananas, peanut butter, cheese, crackers, nuts or dried fruit.

Baby name inspiration

Action movie stars. I'm thinking Vin, Jason, Uma, Tom, Scarlett, Bruce and, of course, Dwayne.

Quiz answers

1. 8 (eight), courtesy of Nadya Suleman in 2009! She had six boys and two girls.
2. The placenta is an organ that develops along with your baby in the uterus during pregnancy. Its job is to pass oxygen and nutrition to the baby from the mother, and to remove waste from their blood, all via the umbilical cord. (I'll be completely honest, this was news to me: before we had a kid I assumed the placenta was a liquid.)
3. True. Studies have been done which showed babies could taste different flavours in the womb - including mint, vanilla and aniseed - based on what their mums had eaten. Don't ask me how those studies were done.
4. They drink it. I'm sorry. They'll grow out of it.
5. False. Those kneecaps don't grow for a while, but when they do, they're adorable.

Week Twelve

Current baby size: Plum
You probably can't tell, but your baby has more than doubled in size over the past three weeks. Talk about aggressive expansion. No one's anywhere near as interested or impressed when I put on weight.

This week's quiz
1. Which side of a woman's brain gets more active during pregnancy - left or right?

2. What is "quickening"?

3. At what time of day does morning sickness typically subside?

4. We know that human babies are born about three months early, and are only totally biologically ready after a full year of pregnancy. Why are they born after nine months?

5. True or false: pregnant women should avoid hot tubs?

A fun activity for this week

If you haven't already, this could be a good week to let your friends, colleagues and wider family know you're expecting a baby. You don't need to make a huge announcement - after all, there's a long way to go in your pregnancy, and you never know what other people are going through. But sharing your good news with people who love you is a wonderful feeling.

Baby name inspiration

The Office. Michael, Jim, Dwight, Pam, Erin, Oscar and so on, if you like the American version. Or David, Tim, Gareth, Dawn and Keith if you prefer the UK version.

Quiz answers

1. The right (creative) side. It's believed this is part of preparing to bond with the baby when they finally arrive.
2. This is the term used to describe the fluttering sensation experienced when your baby begins to move and kick. Quickening typically happens between about 17 and 20 weeks of pregnancy.
3. There is no 'usual' time, unfortunately. You might be fortunate and only have it for a couple of hours (whether that be in morning, afternoon or night) or if you're one of the unfortunate ones, it might be basically constant.
4. The pelvis is too small to pass the head of a baby gestated for a full year, so evolution has led to babies being born at nine months.
5. True, due to increased risk of neural tube defects in your baby.

Week Thirteen

Current baby size: Lemon

You're nearly a third of the way through your pregnancy. It may not have been a breeze so far, but it should be about to get better - the second trimester doesn't get its reputation for being the friendliest trimester for nothing. It's also around this time that your pregnancy starts to feel a little bit more real. There's a visible baby bump. You might have told friends and colleagues. You may have even set eyes on your little one at your first scan. It's all coming together!

This week's quiz

1. It's not proven whether "baby brain" is a thing or not, but what percentage of women report some form of memory impairment during or immediately after pregnancy?

2. Which country produces twins at the highest rate?

3. True or false: babies are born with full-size eyes and 20/20 vision?

4. You'll normally have been given your due date by now, but what percentage of post-term pregnancies are estimated to have been incorrectly dated from the start?

5. And what percentage of babies are actually born on their due date?

A fun activity for this week
Have fun, hypothetical conversations about how you'll parent. What do you want to try to teach your child early? What family traditions might you start? What will you do when they're naughty? Everything you discuss idealistically right now will of course fall by the wayside as soon as your baby is here and you realise the loftiest goal you have is to get them to sleep and eat enough to survive on a daily basis.

Baby name inspiration
Old-school *Thomas the Tank Engine*. I'm talking Edward, Henry, Gordon, James, Percy, Donald, Douglas, Annie and Clarabel. Oh, and Thomas.

Quiz answers
1. 80%. It's not exactly clear what might cause this - it *could* be baby brain, or it could be the cocktail of exhaustion, late nights and the general stress of worrying about a newborn.
2. Benin, at 27.9 per 1,000 births. Who knew?
3. False. Their eyesight develops quite quickly, but they can't see very well at first.
4. About 70%. So don't fixate on that magic due date too much!
5. About 5%. Babies are notoriously unpunctual.

The Second Trimester

The first sequel to the original trimester generally earns more favourable reviews compared to its blockbuster predecessor.

The second trimester, aka the honeymoon period, is also the one in which you actually begin to process the fact that you're going to have a baby. If you're anything like me, that probably means a few late nights spent Googling phrases like 'how to pick up a baby' and 'how to know when to stop feeding a baby'.

It's also when you start to realise your life will never be the same again, so it's a good time to stretch your legs. Get out there and enjoy not being a parent. Your time won't be your own for much longer. If you're pregnant you won't be able to drink and eat certain things, but it's the perfect time to try restaurants, trips and other travels that might not be as simple after your firstborn has arrived.

Week Fourteen

Current baby size: Peach
Your baby is now working hard on their range of facial expressions, giving little smiles and frowns smiling in equal measure.

The expressions aren't really a reflection of their mood: they're just using the muscles and, to some extent, keeping themselves occupied. There's not much to do in the uterus unfortunately, and the WiFi signal is terrible.

This week's quiz
1. Statistically speaking, are you more likely to have a boy or a girl?

2. True or false: pregnant women are less susceptible to broken bones?

3. What is the most common eye colour in newborn babies?

4. At what point do babies start being able to hear?

5. True or false: it is impossible to overfeed a breastfed baby?

A fun activity for this week

Get your house professionally cleaned. You're in the middle of a tough spell; a million things to do and less energy with which to do them all. So take a load off by hiring a cleaner to come in and blitz some of the housework for a change, and do something relaxing instead.

Baby name inspiration

Twilight characters. There's a decent list to go at: Edward, Bella, Jacob, Rosalie, Jasper, Esme, Emmett, Embry and Cora, for example. But personally I was always Team Quil.

Quiz answers

1. A boy. As of 2021, the standard ratio appears to be about 105 boys to every 100 girls.
2. False - they're actually more susceptible due to the presence of joint-softening hormone relaxin.
3. Blue. Their eye colour will change a lot for the first while though, so what they're born with isn't necessarily final.
4. Around week 16 of pregnancy.
5. True. It takes a lot of effort for babies to breastfeed - much more than to bottle feed - so if they don't need to eat, they won't bother.

Week Fifteen

Current baby size: Apple

The whole pregnancy thing should be getting a little easier at this stage. Generally the second trimester is a lot more enjoyable than the first (and the third, come to that), and with the disappearance of morning sickness and other early symptoms, you can look forward to a more comfortable next few months.

This week's quiz

1. What is the world record for the shortest labour?

2. And what is the record for the longest labour?

3. Based on the author's personal experience, where on the changing mat should you position your baby when changing their nappy?

4. Once they're born, approximately how much weight will your baby put on per day during their first month?

5. True or false: when your baby's umbilical stump eventually falls off, it's normal to see a bit of blood around it?

A fun activity for this week

Take a nature hike. Now that there's a little less nausea in the mix, take a walk along a local trail. Nothing too strenuous, but get out for some fresh air and reconnect with nature.

Baby name inspiration

Marvel's *Avengers*. You've got Steve, Tony, Bruce, Clint, Natasha, Scott, Thor, Wanda and Vision to name but a few.

Quiz answers

1. An astounding two minutes, by Australia's Mary Gorgens. She's known as the queen of fast labours and with good reason: she's had five other children, none of whom took longer than two hours deliver, and three of whom were each out in under fifteen minutes!
2. 75 days! In 2012, Joanna Krzysztonek was in her fifth month expecting triplets, when one of them was born prematurely and sadly didn't survive. However, that was medically deemed to be the official start of her labour for all three babies, and after two months the other two arrived safe and well.
3. In the middle of the mat, with their head quite close to the top. My son has a habit of delivering a second wave of projectile poop during a dirty nappy change which has compromised at least one Mitchell family rug when he's been positioned closer to the bottom of the mat, so keeping your baby nice and high will help to catch any surprise deposits.
4. About one ounce (30 grams) per day.
5. True. It's nothing to worry about.

Week Sixteen

Current baby size: Avocado
Wondering when that little baby bump is going to look a bit more pronounced? It may be reasonably soon, as your baby is about to hit a big old growth spurt. Mum may also be able to feel them kicking from this week too - although it's also totally normal you don't feel anything for a little while yet.

This week's quiz
1. Based on the author's experience, which three items are essential for changing your baby's nappy after you've placed them down on the mat?

2. What disease becomes a possibility if a pregnant woman has a negative blood type, but her baby has a positive blood type?

3. If a baby's mother has a negative blood type, and their father has a negative blood type, will the baby's blood type be negative too?

4. True or false: your baby can hiccup in the womb?

5. Should you have a flu jab while pregnant?

A fun activity for this week

Stock up on card games and board games. They're a nice, easy way to while away an afternoon or evening (as long as you and/or your partner aren't too competitive) without going too far.

Baby name inspiration

British monarchs. Think Henry, Elizabeth, James, Anne, George, Mary, Charles, Victoria…

Quiz answers

1. A nappy bag (open it before doing anything else), wipes and the new nappy. It's also a good idea to have easy access to a change of clothes and a muslin square in case your baby produces any unexpected emissions during the change.
2. Rhesus disease. This is harmless to the mother, but in their baby it can lead to anaemia and jaundice. Mothers for whom rhesus disease is a possibility are offered an "anti-d" injection which helps to remove the affected red blood cells before they can cause a problem. If both mother and baby have a negative blood type, rhesus disease is not a possibility.

3. Yes. Although, as my wife and I found out ourselves when discussing rhesus disease with our practitioner, hospitals are not be able to make medical decisions based on a mother-to-be's assertion that a certain person is the father, simply because they wouldn't be the first person to be incorrect about the fact. My wife assured me this is standard practice and not just something they decided to do in her case specifically.

4. True. These will just feel like little belly spasms if you're the person carrying - it's a bit weird but perfectly normal.

5. It's completely up to you. In pregnancy your immune system becomes suppressed, which can make you vulnerable to infections that can complicate your pregnancy. In the UK, the NHS recommends all pregnant women have the seasonal flu jab, but of course it is ultimately your decision. If you have questions or concerns, your midwife or practitioner will be able to help.

Week Seventeen

Current baby size: Pear
Here's a fact that, in my case, really made it sink in that my wife was growing an actual human: in week 17, your baby's hands and feet will develop the swirls and dimples that make up their own unique fingerprints and toe prints. They're getting nearer and nearer to their own little identity. Maybe a few weeks from now they'll get their own driver's licence.

This week's quiz
1. True or false: your baby will soon begin to sneeze inside of the womb?

2. There are six main reasons a newborn baby might cry. How many can you name?

3. Are newborn babies born short-sighted or long-sighted?

4. What is cluster feeding?

5. True or false: red is the first colour babies are able to recognise?

A fun activity for this week

Go for a swim with your partner. Swimming is seen as pretty much the safest exercise you can do while pregnant, and a great way to cool down if you or your partner are running a little hot.

Baby name inspiration

The original Power Rangers. I'm talking Jason, Kimberley, Billy, Trini, Zack and Tommy. Plus Bulk, Skull and Lord Zedd, as well as Zordon, if you're happy to consider the wider cast.

Quiz answers

1. False. They may do a fair bit of hiccuping though!
2. The theory goes that your baby might cry because:

- They're hungry
- They have a full nappy
- They just want to be held (we've all been there)
- They're tired and want to sleep or rest
- They're too hot or too cold
- They don't feel well (or have colic)

I can however confirm from bitter experience that sometimes your baby will be crying and you'll have no real idea why, even after running through the above checklist. Sorry about that.

3. Short-sighted, about 20cm to 30cm in front of them. Makes sense, of course - they can't see very far ahead of them in the womb.

4. It's when babies group their feeds together at specific times of day, increasing the time between feeds at other times of day. It often occurs in the evenings and can be followed by a longer-than-usual period of shuteye, as though your baby is carb-loading for a sleep marathon!

5. True. It's the one that can be most easily processed by their developing eyes.

Week Eighteen

Current baby size: Bell pepper
Here's something adorable: your baby is now yawning. Don't worry, it's not a reflection on your stimulating conversational skills; it's all part of their development.

If you're really lucky, you might just catch a glimpse of it on your next scan. Yes, it's strange to be excited by the sight of a yawn, but that's what we're dealing with here.

This week's quiz
1. What is the usual rule of thumb for knowing how many layers of clothing your baby should be wearing at any given time?

2. How often will a newborn baby wake in the night?

3. What is an 'en caul birth'?

4. What does the word 'placenta' mean in Latin?

5. True or false: changes in the colour of your baby's poop should be a cause for concern?

A fun activity for this week

Read a book. It doesn't have to be about babies, pregnancy or parenting: it can be a violent thriller if that's what you're into. When you're managing a baby 24/7 a few short months from now, you'll yearn for a lazy Sunday spent buried in a story while relaxing in a hot bath, or your bed at midday. Take advantage of it. I'm so jealous that you have the time to read this.

Baby name inspiration

Hamilton. Think Alexander, Eliza, Aaron, Angelica, Hercules, Maria, Thomas, Lafayette… And Peggy.

Quiz answers

1. The typical rule is that they should wear one more layer than you.
2. Generally every two to three hours. This is usually so that they can feed, as their stomachs are still so small.
3. This is where the baby is born still inside their amniotic sac. It's rare, but it happens, and it's totally fine and normal.
4. "Flat cake", in reference to the placenta's pancake-like shape.
5. False. Baby poop changes colour pretty much constantly, but for the most part it's fine and totally normal.

Week Nineteen

Current baby size: Heirloom tomato
Seen your wrinkled fingertips after twenty minutes in the bath and worried about how your baby will look after nine months in amniotic fluid? Fear not. Your baby's skin is now covered in vernix caseosa, a sort of waxy, white coating that kind of laminates their skin while they're still being baked.

Think of it as a cheese-based varnish, provided that thought doesn't completely gross you out.

This week's quiz
1. How many calories per day does breastfeeding burn?

2. How long per day will a 3-month-old usually cry for?

3. For their first 48-72 hours, how many wet nappies (i.e. wee-only) will your baby produce daily?

4. From five days old onwards, how many wet nappies can you expect from them per day?

5. True or false: a newborn baby's head accounts for approximately 10% of their body weight?

A fun activity for this week

It's a good time to discuss and write down your birth plan, so that everyone involved knows what you want on the day, including where you want to be - at home, at hospital, in a birthing pool, and so on.

For my wife and I, the general theme of the plan was essentially "Get the baby out safely, and do whatever the medical experts recommend in order to make that happen", but if you don't want specific pain relief or you want particular things to happen immediately after your baby is delivered, your birth plan is the best place to record it.

Baby name inspiration

Anchorman. I'm thinking Ron, Veronica, Champ, Brian and Brick. Maybe even Wes, if you're an ardent Mantooth fan.

Quiz answers

1. 500. More than some trips to the gym!
2. About one hour. Any more than this and it's best to seek a medical opinion in case there's an underlying cause.
3. Generally two or three.
4. At least six, and they'll be heavy ones.
5. False. It's more like 25%!

Week Twenty

Current baby size: Banana

Welcome to week twenty - AKA the halfway point of your pregnancy. It was around this time that my wife and I found out the gender of our baby (via a note slipped into an envelope by the sonographer, as I wasn't allowed in the scan for pandemic-related reasons). Have you decided whether you're going to find out?

This week's quiz

1. It's around now that you will have the opportunity to find out the gender of your baby, but how accurate are gender ultrasounds thought to be?

2. The average woman's skin surface measures around 17 square feet when she's not pregnant. How much skin surface does she have by the last week of her pregnancy?

3. What is a good rule of thumb for how many dirty nappies (i.e. poopy) nappies to expect from your baby in the first four days after they're born?

4. You might find that it helps to soothe your baby to sleep when they're swaddled, but should you put your baby down to sleep at night while swaddled?

5. By what stage should you have the house fully 'childproofed'?

A fun activity for this week
Now that you've had your 20-week scan and potentially know the gender of your baby, you might want to start picking up particular clothes and refining that all-important name list!

Baby name inspiration
Billionaires. My personal favourites are Elon, Bill, Bernard, Mark, Mackenzie, Julia, Warren, Larry, Jacqueline, Gina and Jeff. But especially Jeff.

Quiz answers
1. Just over 98% accurate. So, good, but not perfect.
2. 18.5 square feet!
3. Normally the amount of dirty nappies will roughly match the number of days old they are - so one dirty nappy on day one, two on day two and so on. Don't worry, the pattern ends long before day one hundred: from four days onwards they'll normally do three or four per day, and by the time they're two or three months old, it'll be one a day, or even every couple of days.

4. Yes and no. It's fine to swaddle them, but it's best to keep their arms free, just in case they happen to roll themselves over in the night.

5. By the time your baby is six months old, at the latest. But there's a lot to do - everything from child locks and stair gates to window guards and plug socket covers - so start as soon as you can, ideally before your baby even arrives.

Week Twenty-One

Current baby size: Papaya
Your baby is growing nicely and packing on a few more pounds. Actually, this point is the first stage at which they've weighed more than the placenta. (The placenta carries on growing throughout the pregnancy, just not as fast as the baby). Anyway, I'll stop going on about your baby's weight. I don't want to make them self-conscious.

This week's quiz
1. True or false: during pregnancy, a female orgasm can induce contractions?

2. When a pregnant woman goes into labour, what comes first: their contractions or their waters breaking?

3. When a pregnant woman's waters do break, what colours should they be?

4. Who has the greater amount of taste buds, an adult or a baby?

5. True or false: if you think your baby has reflux, you should prop up the head of their Moses basket or cot to help ease it?

A fun activity for this week
Find a forest and go for a nice walk together. Enjoy the range of motion while you can. Once you reach the third trimester it will become a lot harder.

Baby name inspiration
Tennis stars past and present. Roger, Serena, Rafael, Tim, Venus, Novak, Maria, Andy, Pete, Billie, Martina, Coco...

Quiz answers
1. True. Essentially, while a male orgasm may have got you into this situation, a female orgasm might get you out of it.
2. This varies from woman to woman. Most of the time contractions start first, but approximately 1 in 15 pregnancies (including my wife) see waters break first - they'll then either go into labour naturally within 48 hours, or will otherwise be induced to get things moving.
3. Clear or pale yellow. You may also find that they're slightly bloodstained at first. If the waters are coloured or smelly, contact your midwife right away, as your baby might be at risk of infection.
4. Perhaps surprisingly, it's a baby. They have around 30,000 taste buds compared to just 10,000 for adults.
5. False. This is not recommended anymore. Reflux will generally go away on its own but see your practitioner if your baby is distressed, or if they have been suffering with it for more than two weeks.

Week Twenty-Two

Current baby size: Grapefruit

At this point in your pregnancy, your baby will be getting into a recognisable routine of sleeping and waking - although sadly it may not be the same as yours. Our first-born would regularly have a little rave in the womb at around 7pm each evening, which was pretty convenient in comparison to a colleague of mine, whose daughter was regularly raising the roof at about 3 o'clock in the morning.

This week's quiz

1. You might feel like your pregnancy still has a long way to go, but what is the longest pregnancy ever recorded?

2. In pregnancy, what are Braxton Hicks?

3. Which item will you generally need before the hospital will allow you to leave with your baby?

4. Which substance is typically used to limit pregnancy stretch marks?

5. What was the birth weight of the heaviest ever newborn?

A fun activity for this week

Arrange a date night or, even better, a "babymoon". Me-time will be in extremely short supply after your baby arrives, but quality us-time will be even rarer. So have a fancy meal or your favourite takeaway, have a big night in watching movies, get out to do something you love together or get away for a week or a weekend. And cuddle up as much as you can. Once your baby is here, cuddling your partner probably isn't going to be very high in your list of priorities. Trust me.

Baby name inspiration

Your favourite boybands and girlbands. The list is endless, but I'll kick you off with Geri, Justin, Perrie, Cheryl, AJ, Nick and Abz.

Quiz answers

1. 375 days, or 53.5 weeks! Baby Penny was (eventually) delivered courtesy of Beulah Hunter in 1945. That length of pregnancy is highly unusual, but many other women have experienced pregnancies lasting 10 or 11 months.
2. They're the name given to when the womb contracts and relaxes during the second or third trimester - they're kind of like the uterus practicing for labour!
3. A car seat.
4. Cocoa butter.
5. 22lbs, 8oz. Good lord.

Week Twenty-Three

Current baby size: Ear of corn

Your baby's lungs aren't yet showing off their full repertoire of abilities, mainly because they're getting all of the oxygen they need from their mum via the placenta - but they are getting in plenty of breathing movement practice to help prepare them for life outside the womb. Don't worry, they'll prove quite quickly how well their lungs work when they're screaming in your face at 2 in the morning.

This week's quiz

1. The amount of blood in a woman's body increases by what percentage during pregnancy?

2. What is an 'assisted delivery'?

3. On average, who spends longer in the womb: baby boys or baby girls?

4. How long on average does it take a baby to double their birth weight?

5. In centimetres, how much will your baby grow in height per month in their first year?

A fun activity for this week

Get booked onto an antenatal class. These courses are a great way to meet other people in the same boat, make new friends and pick up some great tips about pregnancy, labour, babies and parenting.

Baby name inspiration

Friends characters. Ross, Rachel, Chandler, Monica, Joey and Phoebe. And Gunther.

Quiz answers

1. 50%. This means a pregnant woman's heart also grows at the same time in order to deliver it around the body.
2. This is essentially when instruments are used to assist the baby out. This may be because of difficulties during the second stage of labour, such as the baby becoming distressed or not being in the right position for delivery, or if the labour has been long and exhaustion is setting in.
3. Apparently, girl babies spend a day longer in the womb on average than boy babies.
4. About five months. It happens *really* stealthily, so that you simply start to worry your arms are getting weaker.
5. About 1cm to 1.5cm. They'd end up taller than a bungalow if they kept that pace up through their life.

Week Twenty-Four

Current baby size: Cantaloupe
This is the point at which your baby's lungs and other vital organs are developed enough for them to have a chance of survival if they were born now. Of course, there are still a lot of risks if your little one was to arrive so prematurely. We want them to stay inside for a decent while yet, so that they're fully-cooked when they emerge!

This week's quiz
1. Suffering from persistent heartburn during your pregnancy might indicate that your baby has a lot of what?

2. Estrogen is the main hormone that helps to protect and grow your baby, and so pregnant women create much more of it than they would normally. How long would it take a non-pregnant woman to produce the same amount of estrogen that a pregnant woman creates in a day?

3. True or false: the baby belly disappears almost immediately after giving birth?

4. True or false: around this stage of pregnancy, it's possible for someone to hear the baby's heartbeat simply by pressing an ear to the bump?

5. When is the best time to put your baby down to sleep?

A fun activity for this week
Figure out your baby's sleeping situation for their first six months. It's highly recommended that they sleep in the same room as you, so it's worth looking at cots, cribs and co-sleeper that attach to the bed to see what's going to work best for you. Do a little bit of measuring and see if you need to move a few things to make it work. My wife and I decided to swap preferred sides of the bed so that our son wouldn't be sleeping on the side nearest the radiator and the window.

Baby name inspiration
Tarantino characters. Mia, Vincent, Jules, Elle, Beatrix, Calvin, Mallory, Budd, Winston, and Mr Blonde.

Quiz answers
1. Hair. It's believed that the same hormones which result in heartburn can also play a role in how much hair babies grow in the womb.
2. A year - and it can be as much as three years at full term!

3. False. Pregnancy is a huge thing for a body to go through and, despite what celebrity post-baby photoshoots might imply, its effects hang around for a long while.

4. True, from about 27 weeks, which is kind of mind-blowing. However in my case it was basically impossible to tell the baby's heartbeat from my wife's, along with everything else going on in there, so you may just have to make an assumption that you've heard it...

5. The trick is to put them in their crib or bed when they're still awake but drowsy, so that they get used to soothing themselves back to sleep, even if they wake up in the night.

Week Twenty-Five

Current baby size: Cauliflower

By now your baby is likely kicking, stretching and pushing a lot. and might even be responding to your touch or even your voice. Our son reacted really strongly to 'Uptown Funk' for some reason, even though he's never shown any interest in it since he was born.

He was also a big hiccuper inside the womb, which is pretty much the cutest thing imaginable when you're resting a hand on him or her, waiting for them to emerge.

This week's quiz

1. How many hours per day does a newborn baby typically sleep?

2. In pregnancy, what is "pica"?

3. Why should you talk to your baby in a higher-pitched voice?

4. How often should you sterilise your baby's bottles?

5. True or false: a newborn baby's cry tends to mimic the language of their mother?

A fun activity for this week

Try playing different types of music to the bump and see if your baby responds. It doesn't have to be 'Uptown Funk', but maybe avoid death metal or anything too hardcore.

Baby name inspiration

US Presidents - imagine introducing friends and family to your little Donald, Barack, George, Bill, Abraham, Richard or Theodore.

Quiz answers

1. 14 to 17 hours. Don't worry if it's less, though. Our son was getting about half that, which is also totally fine and normal.
2. It's the term given to cravings for things that aren't supposed to be eaten - chalk, burnt matches, soap, sand and so on.
3. There are quite a few reasons - the sing-songy style is easier for your baby to follow, lets them know that what you're saying is directed at them, and generally helps them to learn language and enunciation. Plus, it sounds funny.
4. After every single use. This is an advantage of breastfeeding - no worrying about sterilising bottles and waiting for them to cool down so that you can use them at all hours.
5. True. So bizarre.

Week Twenty-Six

Current baby size: Lettuce
If you could see your baby's eyes at this stage, you'd be able to see that they're now open, and it won't be long until they start practicing their blinking. This explains why my son was born with the ability to wink like a flirtatious colonel.

Every baby's eyes tend to be blue at this stage in a pregnancy, but that will change both before and after they're born. They'll have settled on a colour by the time your baby is about three years old.

This week's quiz
1. You'll need to properly sterilise all of your baby's feeding equipment to make sure all germs are killed. What is the temperature needed to eradicate harmful bacteria?

2. How old should your baby be before you feed them cow's milk or honey?

3. How long should you let your newborn cry for before attending to them?

4. Which way do 85% of babies prefer to turn their heads when lying on their backs?

5. True or false: worldwide, more babies are born on Tuesdays than on any other day?

A fun activity for this week

Get batch-cooking and freezing some delicious meals so that you have some quick, nutritious options to heat up when you're busy looking after a newborn. We filled our freezer with bolognese, chilli con carne, stew and a wide range of curries, and each one was like a little takeaway from the past. It's easy to forget to eat in those early days, and you need to keep your energy up more than ever, so make life easy for yourself.

Baby name inspiration

Characters in Shakespeare plays. The likes of Rosalind, Iago, Ophelia, Romeo, Portia, Duncan, Horatio, Ariel, Toby and Viola might appeal.

Quiz answers

1. 80°C (176°F).

2. At least one year old. Honey carries certain bacterias that are unfriendly to very young babies, and they struggle to digest cow's milk.

3. You should pick them up immediately. Before I became a parent, I assumed you needed to leave babies for a certain amount of time to see if they soothed themselves. However, it turns out babies are pretty basic, primal creatures - if they're crying, it's because they need something.

4. To the right. This might be linked to the fact that more people are right-handed too.

5. True! Perhaps Pancake Day helps to tip the balance.

Week Twenty-Seven

Current baby size: Cucumber

As your baby continues to grow and pack on muscle and fat, they'll start to feel a bit cramped in the uterus. That's nothing to worry about - there's still plenty of room for them to grow into. It does mean though that their little kicks, wriggles and somersaults will reduce or become a little softer as their limbs get more restricted. They'll make up for it once they're in your arms.

This week's quiz

1. Most nappies now have a strip on the front which changes colour when your baby wets it. What colour will it be if your baby has a wet nappy?

2. Babies cannot taste salt until they are how old?

3. How many days of sleep do babies deprive their parents of in their first year?

4. When can you begin to introduce your baby to solid foods?

5. True or false: until your baby is a toddler, they can only sleep with one pillow in their cot?

A fun activity for this week

Join a group for parents-to-be, either in person or on video calls. It's fun to talk to people at the same stage you're at, and you can share a lot of useful information and provide a sounding board for one another.

Baby name inspiration

Peep Show characters. If my wife and I have another six children, I'll probably be pushing to name them Mark, Jeremy, Sophie, Big Suze, Super Hans and Mad Andy.

Quiz answers

1. Blue.
2. Four months. This is thought to be due to the timing of their kidney development.
3. 44 days! Get your sleep while you can.
4. At around 4 to 6 months old.
5. False - your baby can't sleep with any pillow at all until they are a toddler, as it increases the risk of SIDS, overheating, suffocation and so on.

The Third Trimester

Aka the trimester in which things get real. Really real.

Are you excited? Or nervous? You're probably a bit of both. You might be two-thirds of the way there, but there's still a long way to go - and a lot of weight for your baby to pack on yet!

One piece of advice I can give you during this last phase of pregnancy is to absorb as much information as you can about looking after an actual newborn.

It's easy to spend the last trimester focusing on the labour and delivery part, and that *is* important, but once you're through it you'll be quickly left to look after a tiny, precious human, which is also important. You'll learn a lot on the job, but a little knowledge to start you off can help a lot.

But you know what? Whatever you do, you'll be great, because you care. You wouldn't be reading this book if you didn't. Your baby is incredibly lucky to have a parent who cares as much as you.

So my other piece of advice is not to worry. Don't beat yourself up when you make mistakes. And don't believe people on social media whose parenting experience appears to be one big, sunny daydream. Every new parent - *every single one* - struggles at times. It's part of what makes it all so worthwhile.

Week Twenty-Eight

Current baby size: Aubergine (or eggplant, depending on which side of the pond you reside)

Your baby's heartbeat is now nice and strong. You'd now be able to hear it through a stethoscope pressed to the bump or even, if you're not the one who's actually pregnant, by placing your ear to it if you can find the right place. As I mentioned earlier, I was only ever able to pick up my wife's heartbeat and general tummy grumblings when I tried this.

With just 12 weeks until your due date, it's also a good time to start making your hospital bag checklist and getting everything packed. It might not be too long now until you need it.

This week's quiz

1. How long should each of your baby's feeds take?

2. Where should you put your baby down to sleep: on their back, front or side?

3. At what age do babies tend to start showing separation anxiety?

4. 75% of women develop a "linea nigra" during pregnancy. What is this?

5. True or false: babies cry in the womb?

A fun activity for this week
Start preparing your baby book or box - an archive of all of the milestones your baby has hit so far, and will go on to hit! It's the perfect way to keep all of those scan photos, hospital wristbands, pregnancy/new baby greetings cards in one place so that you can reminisce over them in the future when your baby isn't so little.

Baby name inspiration
Weather. Rain, Gale, Storm, Misty, Coro and Talia are all weather-inspired names in one way or another. Seasons are also growing in popularity, with Summer, Autumn and Winter all strong choices. I'm not sure why Spring has never taken off in the same way.

Quiz answers
1. There's no real right answer to this. This important thing is actually not to time the feeds if you can help it, as your baby will feed for as long as they need to, to get the amount of milk or formula they need. Sometimes it may take 10 minutes, other times it may be 20 minutes or more.

2. Their back, as the chance of SIDS is higher for babies who are sometimes placed on their front or side.

3. Around seven months. Don't worry, they usually get more chilled about this by the time they're two years old...

4. It's the dark line that runs vertically down the middle of the stomach.

5. Amazingly, this is true! Scientists have found that babies begin to cry silently in the womb during the third trimester. It's believed to be a practice for the real thing, rather than a reaction to anything. Remember, crying and looking cute are basically babies' only two survival tactics initially.

Week Twenty-Nine

Current baby size: Coconut
No doubt your baby will be continuing to make their presence known at this stage, and you'll have a good idea of their routine by now. Every pregnancy and every baby are different, so there's no set number or pattern of movements you should be looking out for. The key thing is to get familiar with what's normal for your baby. If their usual pattern changes, you should contact your midwife or hospital.

This week's quiz
1. According to the NHS, 60% of pregnant women experience carpal tunnel syndrome as a result of fluid build-up in their tissue, particularly during the third trimester. Where will they feel tingling and numbness as a sign of this?

2. And how long after giving birth might a woman continue to feel those pins and needles?

3. To the nearest hundred, approximately how many nappies will your baby get through in their first year?

4. True or false: babies can breathe and swallow at the same time?

5. What is delayed cord-clamping?

A fun activity for this week
Make a baby item wishlist on Amazon or similar. For one thing, it's useful to see what you still need to get. For another, you will likely get asked by friends and family what you would like as a gift, and you don't want to receive six identical bumbos or similar, so it helps to be able to direct people to a list of things you want and don't have yet.

Baby name inspiration
Motown legends. I'll kick you off with Marvin, Diana, Smokey, Stevie, Lionel, Al, Tammi and Gladys.

Quiz answers
1. In their hands and fingers.
2. Up to six weeks.
3. 3400. And don't even get me started on the amount of wipes.
4. True. This is because to begin with their larynx sits up high in the nasal cavity like a snorkel!

5. Cutting the umbilical cord immediately after the baby is born has been routine practice for years. However more recent research has suggested that cutting the cord too early may mean that the baby misses out on nutrients from the blood. This has created a modern preference for delaying clamping and cutting until after the cord has stopped passing on its good stuff, provided there is no medical reason to speed things up.

Week Thirty

Current baby size: Broccoli

Congratulation, you're officially three quarters of the way to your baby's due date! Ten weeks will still feel like such a long time, but it will likely begin to pass quickly now as your hospital check-ups become more frequent. In the meantime, your baby's sucking reflex is taking shape around nicely - no they're practicing on their fingers and thumbs in preparation for that first feed from you or your partner.

This week's quiz

1. How much weight is your baby putting on each week at this stage?

2. What is lanugo?

3. When cleaning up a baby girl after a number two, which way should you wipe: front-to-back or back-to-front?

4. Approximately what temperature should a room be in which your baby sleeps?

5. And roughly what temperature should your baby's bath water be?

A fun activity for this week

Get your baby's medical kit ready. Gripe water, Infacol, Calpol, a baby thermometer, tiny nail clippers and so on. You won't use most of this in the first few months, but it's best to have it there ready when you need it.

Baby name inspiration

American Idol winners. Laine, Maddie, Trent, Caleb, Candice, Kris, Carrie, Ruben and, of course, Kelly.

Quiz answers

1. Half a pound every week. And you'll celebrate every single ounce.
2. The coat of downy hair that covers your baby to keep them warm. Don't worry, they'll generally shed most of this before birth, although some are born still wearing it!
3. Front to back, to avoid any nasty little UTIs.
4. Between 16°C and 20°C.
5. About 38°C - around body temperature.

Week Thirty-One

Current baby size: Cabbage

Sleeping with a bump can be very tricky at this stage. It might be useful to invest in a pregnancy pillow if you haven't already. Equally, you might find that the best thing is to gather all of the pillows and cushions in the house and make a little maternity nest.

This week's quiz

1. Around this stage a pregnant woman may notice the baby's first milk leaking from their nipples. What is this first nutrient-rich milk known as?

2. During labour, a woman's cervix needs to dilate by what amount (in cm) to accommodate the baby's head?

3. What is colic and what causes it in babies?

4. True or false: Some babies are born with teeth?

5. And when will your baby typically sprout their first tooth?

A fun activity for this week

Get your baby's newborn clothes organised. You'll need to wash them before they first get worn, so dedicating a day or two to some advance baby laundry, and then putting the clothes away in an orderly way that will make it easy for you to grab the right sizes when you need them, will pay dividends. You'll probably find you'll do a lot of baby-changing in your general living area, not just in the nursery, so it's worth having clean, available clothes in both places.

Baby name inspiration

Tekken characters. Think Nina, Marshall, Lee, Eddy, Paul, Lili, Jack, King and Yoshimitsu.

Quiz answers

1. Colostrum.
2. 10cm. Oof.
3. Colic is effectively when your baby is crying a lot for no apparent reason. You'll hear parents and grandparents talk about it from time to time, but no one knows for sure why it happens - it's really weird. Some experts think it may be linked to digestion, but right now, medically, it's kind of a symptom (a lot of crying) with no cause.
4. True. Which might sound horrifying, but it's fine and very cute.
5. When they're around 5-7 months old.

Week Thirty-Two

Current baby size: Squash

This week the quiz focuses on pain relief options during labour - it's worth both parties thinking about these early so that you can express your preferences to your care team.

This week's quiz

1. What is Entonox better known as?

2. How long does it take Entonox to take effect?

3. What is TENS, as a pain relief option?

4. Pethidine or diamorphine is injected into the muscle in your arm or leg to offer mild pain relief, but what is a possible risk of pethidine or diamorphine to your baby?

5. How long does an epidural take to work?

A fun activity for this week

Take a practice run over to the hospital you're expecting your baby to be born in, if you haven't already done so.

Even if you know where it is, try a few different routes in case there's a diversion or other issue on the day, and suss out the parking situation so that you have at least five alternate options to try in case it happens to be crowded. Also, make sure you have plenty of change in the car if it's a paid parking situation.

Baby name inspiration

Succession characters. Logan, Kendall, Roman, Connor, Siobhan, Tom and Gregory. I mean, who wouldn't want to be a part of the Roy family?

Quiz answers

1. Gas and air, or nitrous oxide, delivered via a mouthpiece.
2. About 20 seconds. The effects wear off after a couple of minutes, so it's usually best for a labouring mother using Entonox to begin taking it on at the first hint of a contraction to help take the edge off of any pain.
3. TENS (transcutaneous electrical nerve stimulation) delivers a gentle electrical current through pads on your back. You control the intensity of the current via a little handset.
4. Pethidine and diamorphine can sometimes make your baby drowsy and slow to breathe when they first arrive.
5. An epidural takes 20 minutes to set up and then another 20 minutes to take effect. It is partly for this reason that epidurals are not recommended late in labour.

Week Thirty-Three

Current baby size: Pineapple

It all probably feels a bit like *Groundhog Day* at the moment. There's still a number of impatient, uncomfortable weeks to spend going around in circles until your due date - and even more if you happen to go overdue.

So the best thing you can do at this point is talk. Talk to everyone. Other parents. Your midwife. Family and friends. Your social media groups. Tap into that support network and put the pregnancy world to rights. It'll help pass the time and put you at ease when you need it most.

This week's quiz

1. Approximately how many times a day will you need to feed your baby for the first two days after birth?

2. And what about over days three to five?

3. What is "engorgement" in baby-feeding terms?

4. Which vegetable is thought to help ease engorgement?

5. What is considered a safe percentage of birth weight for a baby to lose in their first week?

A fun activity for this week
Have a few dry runs at sterilising dummies, bottles, pump equipment and anything else you'll regularly need to clean, with whichever method/s you've elected to use. It's also worth having a practice at making up some formula. Even if you're planning to breastfeed your baby, it's useful to have an alternative and know how to use it, just in case.

Baby name inspiration
Stranger Things characters - for example, Dustin, Eleven, Mike, Will, Lucas, Nancy, Steve, Joyce and Demogorgon.

Quiz answers
1. About six times per day, roughly every two to three hours.
2. Eight to twelve times per day.
3. It is the term given to when a breastfeeding mother's breasts fill up with milk, becoming uncomfortably firm, heavy and sore.
4. Cabbage leaves. Apparently they contain an enzyme that acts as an anti-inflammatory.
5. 10%.

Week Thirty-Four

Current baby size: Butternut squash

By now your baby has pretty much reached their birth height - although you wouldn't know it from the way they're curled up with their knees tucked into their chest. Their legs will stay folded up like this for a little while, but it's totally normal. It does though mean that, when they start to straighten them, it seems like they've doubled in length overnight.

This week's quiz

1. Babies usually lose weight after they first arrive. When do most of them regain their birth weight?

2. What is a 'ventouse' birth?

3. At what age will your baby likely take their first step?

4. And at what age can babies usually understand basic words such as "No" and "Bye Bye"?

5. True or false: babies have the ability to smell while still in the womb?

A fun activity for this week

Set up your changing station/s (for ease you'll want the station/s near to where the baby sleeps overnight and to where they spend most of their waking hours) and stock them up with nappies, wipes, nappy bags, nappy bin and so on. Practice the motions of changing a nappy or two to make sure the feng shui's all right,

Baby name inspiration

Former Oasis band members. Liam, Noel, Tony, Alan, Paul, Zak, Gem, Andy and Bonehead.

Quiz answers

1. Between two and three weeks old.
2. Sometimes medical intervention is required during labour. A ventouse (or vacuum extraction) has a suction cup that is attached to the baby's head during labour and is held in place by a vacuum created by a pump. It has a handle, which is used to ease the baby down the birth canal as you push. A baby delivered by ventouse will have a 'cone-shaped' head, but this will disappear soon after delivery.
3. Nine to twelve months.
4. Around nine months.
5. True. As they breathe in the amniotic fluid, this helps them to become familiar with their mother's scent.

Week Thirty-Five

Current baby size: Romaine lettuce
By this week, it's more than likely your baby has moved into eject-ready position, with their head pointing downwards towards the cervix. This is partly because it's the most comfortable way for them to fit in what is by now a very cramped uterus. Think of it as them having arrived in the departure lounge. Now they're just waiting for boarding.

This week's quiz
1. When can you expect to see your baby smile for the first time?

2. At what age will you be able to give your baby a pacifier or dummy?

3. And by which age should you remove a pacifier or dummy from their routine?

4. In pregnancy, what is 'lightening'?

5. And what is a 'Lotus birth'?

A fun activity for this week

I use the term 'fun' loosely here, but it's good to do some admin prep for after your baby arrives. Research kids' bank accounts, how to get a birth certificate, government child support and how to register your little one for things like the doctor or dentist.

Baby name inspiration

Harry Potter. You've got Harry, of course, but Hermione, Ron, Fred, Ginny, Lily and little Voldemort are similarly compelling options.

Quiz answers

1. Between six and eight weeks, once their facial muscles have developed enough. At first, it'll probably be wind, but they'll soon be grinning when they see you.
2. Three to four weeks.
3. By four years old at the absolute latest, your baby should have moved on from using their pacifier. This helps to reduce the risk of ear infections, yeast infections and other conditions.
4. Lightening is where the baby drops and settles into the mother's pelvis late in the third trimester, as they prepare to make their grand entrance.

5. This is where parents choose to leave the placenta attached to the baby, believing that it continues to provide nourishment until it drops off on its own. It's not very common practice to choose this, and some hospitals won't even allow you to do it.

Week Thirty-Six

Current baby size: Swiss chard

Another milestone - by the end of this week, you'll be in your last month of pregnancy! Don't cheer too loudly though, because your baby's ears are now more sensitive than ever - to the point that they might be able to recognise your voice and particular sounds after they're born.

This week's quiz

1. How many bones will your baby be born with?

2. True or false: when newborns cry, they don't produce tears?

3. True or false: the brains of newborn boys grow faster than the brains of newborn girls?

4. Should you sleep your newborn baby on their side, back or front?

5. Which month of the year sees the birth of the heaviest babies on average?

A fun activity for this week
Practice fitting the car seat - as in, fitting it into the car, and adjusting the straps to fit a baby securely into it. If you don't happen to have a spare/volunteer baby around, make yourself a towel baby (Google it if you've not come across towel babies before) and use that. The first time I tried to adjust my car seat was literally when I was fumbling about to put my 4-day-old son into it when bringing him home from the hospital, which I wouldn't recommend if you want to retain the respect of your children.

Baby name inspiration
Super Bowl MVPs. Julian, Eli, Peyton, Dexter, Kurt, Troy and Ottis. Some rookie named Tom has won it a bit too.

Quiz answers
1. About 300, about 94 more than you and I (unless you happen to be a baby yourself), but, as they grow, some of those bones will fuse together, leaving them with the standard 206 or so.
2. True! So don't worry, this isn't a sign they're dehydrated. (A friend of ours didn't know this and freaked out when she first realised her baby wasn't producing tears whenever he cried.)
3. True. This mainly happens over the first three months, and the part of the brain that controls coordination grows particularly fast in newborn boys compared to newborn girls.
4. You should place them down to sleep on their back.

5. May. Apologies if your due date falls in that month...

Week Thirty-Seven

Current baby size: Honeydew melon

Welcome to month nine of your pregnancy. Nearly there now! At 37 weeks, your pregnancy is considered full-term. Your baby is ready to be born, and you'll be meeting them in the next few weeks. Rest up and sleep as much as you can for this last period, because life is about to change!

This week's quiz

1. Once your baby is born, should you try keep their umbilical cord stump dry, or moist?

2. As your baby is born, you may notice that they have a 'caput'. What is a caput?

3. Which babies are likely to be heavier at birth - boys or girls?

4. What is a foetal scalp electrode?

5. What percentage of your newborn's height will their head account for?

A fun activity for this week

Pick out and pack your baby's going-home outfit. This isn't really about what'll look best on the 'gram. You'll want a soft, easy-to-put-on (i.e. doesn't need to go over their head) outfit which isn't too baggy so that they'll fit snugly in the car seat without their clothing getting pushed up over their face.

Baby name inspiration

Academy Award nominated directors. Clint, Ridley, Kathryn, Sofia, Warren, Greta, Mel, Adam, Jordan, Quentin and Ang.

Quiz answers

1. Dry. It's best not to bath then until after the cord has dropped off of its own, well, accord.
2. It's the term given to the more elongated head shape your baby might emerge with having passed through the birth canal. Don't worry, it's only temporary while their skull plates harden.
3. Boys. The theory goes that women carrying boys are likely to eat more during pregnancy. That said, my son was expected to be pretty big (based mainly on the midwife grasping my wife's bump during a couple of third trimester check-ups), had a growth scan at 38 weeks where the hospital estimated him to be at least 8lbs, and was then born two weeks later at 7lbs 1, so you can't read too much into this.

4. This is where a small clip is placed on the baby's scalp during labour to directly monitor their heart rate. It'll leave them with a little bit of a scratch on their head but it can mean the medical team have better visibility of what's going on. Ultimately it's your choice whether you let them do this.

5. About 25%. In adults it's more like 15%. I don't want to get too scientific but, relatively speaking, babies have big old heads and tiny bodies.

Week Thirty-Eight

Current baby size: Pumpkin
You're bearing down on your due date now, but remember, 95% of babies don't arrive on their due date. 25% come early and 70% come late. So basically, be continually ready to go, day or night, over the next four weeks!

This week's quiz
1. Once you get into the routine of having your baby's height and weight measured, you'll become very aware of which 'percentile' they fall into versus other children of the same age and gender. Which child is bigger, one in the 5th percentile, or one in the 95th percentile?

2. Your placenta weighs what proportion of your baby's birth weight?

3. What does it mean if a baby is 'breech'?

4. An epidural is a local anaesthetic given to numb the nerves during labour. Where on the mother's body is an epidural delivered?

5. Are you allowed to take paracetamol or any other over-the-counter painkiller during your labour?

A fun activity for this week
Start browsing for some books you might like to read your baby as they grow. Everything from Spot the Dog and the Gruffalo to Harry Potter. It's a good time to practice your storybook voices too - your baby will love to hear you bring characters to life!

Baby name inspiration
Fifty Shades of Grey. Some classics here. Anastasia, Christian, Jack, Jason, Elena, Elliot, Katherine, Grace, Mia, Leila and Jose, to name but a few.

Quiz answers
1. The 95th percentile. The higher the percentile number, the bigger a baby is, versus kids of the same age and gender.
2. About one-sixth.
3. Your baby is in the breech position if they're lying bottom or feet first in the uterus, as opposed to head down. If this is the case at 36 weeks, your medical team will discuss safe deliver options with you.
4. The back. Due to the effectiveness of this method, it can make it difficult for a woman to push and may require the use of forceps.
5. Yes.

Week Thirty-Nine

Current baby size: Watermelon
Getting sudden bursts of energy to tidy and organise things? It might be your nesting instinct kicking in, which some believe is a sign of imminent labour. My wife went on an uncharacteristic cleaning spree the weekend of our week 39, and then her waters broke later the same night, so I do wonder if there's something in this.

This week's quiz
1. During birth, what is delivered first, the baby or the placenta?

2. What is usually the first injection offered to a newborn baby soon after birth?

3. What is apparently the only scientifically-proven method for bringing on labour during pregnancy?

4. True or false: You should never wake a sleeping baby?

5. What vitamin supplement is it recommended that breastfed babies take daily throughout their first year?

A fun activity for this week

Can't wait until your due date? Try what many consider to be the holy trinity of inducing labour naturally: curry, sex and lot of walking. (Not simultaneously, obviously.)

Baby name inspiration

The UK version of *Gladiators*. This might seem a niche seam to mine, but I invite you to consider Ace, Jet, Hunter, Blaze, Rio, Wolf, Falcon and Zodiac.

Quiz answers

1. The baby.
2. Vitamin K. This is to prevent a rare bleeding disorder called HDN. You can have them take it orally if you'd prefer, but they'll need follow-up doses.
3. Nipple stimulation. It seems that it triggers the release of oxytocin to start one's contractions. This is also known as the "comfort technique".
4. False. For example, if it's been a while since your baby was fed and it's time for them to feed again, you should (gently) wake them. Occasionally that sleepiness can be a sign that they're dehydrated.
5. Vitamin D. The best source of it is sunlight on the skin, but you have to be extremely careful to protect your baby's skin in the sun, hence the supplement.

Week Forty

Current baby size: Roughly the size of a newborn baby

The final countdown has very much begun by this point. Unfortunately it's a countdown that may well carry on past the date you've been counting down to. Our son actually arrived the day before his due date, which seems insanely punctual compared to some of the stories you hear (and considering how terrible his parents' time-keeping is). Almost there now!

This week's quiz

1. While breastfeeding, how often should a new mother wash her breasts?

2. When will your baby's umbilical stump fall off?

3. What is a membrane sweep, and why might one be suggested to you?

4. When can you first give your baby a bath?

5. And how often will you give your baby a bath in his or her first 6 months?

A fun activity for this week

Refresh your stocks of contraception. You likely won't be in the mood for sex immediately after the birth, but when you eventually are, you'll be very fertile so it's best to be prepared!

Baby name inspiration

Schitt's Creek. Top seven options being David, Patrick, Alexis, Ted, Moira, Johnny and Roland.

Quiz answers

1. It's actually better not to wash them, as this dulls the Montgomery tubercles (the little raised bumps on the areola) which secrete an oil to protect the nipple for breastfeeding, and also help attract the baby to latch. Relatedly, 'The Montgomery Tubercles' will likely be the name of my street poetry collective.
2. One to two weeks following birth. Just don't do anything with it (don't clean it or get it wet) and let it fall off naturally.
3. If your baby is past due date or needs to come early, you may be offered a membrane sweep as a drug-free way of encouraging labour. This is where your midwife will insert a finger into the cervix and try to separate the sac surrounding your baby from it. After a membrane sweep, labour often starts within 48 hours.
4. The World Health Organisation recommends waiting until at least 24 hours after birth, but it's best to stick to sponge baths until the umbilical stump has fallen off.
5. No more than three times per week. Once a week is actually fine.

Weeks Forty-One & Forty-Two

Current baby size: A slightly bigger and more impatient newborn baby than last week

If you've made it this far, the end is in sight. By the time you reach this stage, you'll normally have an induction booked in already, so you'll know roughly when you'll be meeting your baby if they don't make an appearance before then. Don't worry, they'll be in your arms soon!

This week's quiz

1. If you're over your due date, you might be heading towards "being induced". What actually happens when a pregnant woman is induced?

2. What percentage of pregnant women have labour induced?

3. What proportion of women give birth via caesarean?

4. What is foetal scalp electrode?

5. Finally, once your baby arrives, how long do you have to register their birth?

A fun activity for this week
While you still have time on your hands, and if you can be bothered, it can be good to get ahead and figure out how to make easy work of sending out thank you cards for all of the well wishes and lovely gifts you'll no doubt be receiving very soon. I downloaded a postcard app that allowed us to drop pictures of our newborn son into some basic templates and write them out online, which made things a lot simpler.

Baby name inspiration
Your family tree. We have a surprising number of Abrahams in ours. My wife and I didn't name our son Abraham, but we might not even have considered doing so otherwise.

Quiz answers
1. Her care team will stimulate her contractions in order to trigger labour, usually by providing her with artificial hormones.
2. Around 20% of pregnant women in the UK have labour induced.
3. One in three – the ratio has actually tripled in the last ten years.
4. A foetal scalp electrode attaches to your baby's head during labour to pick up their heartbeat directly.
5. Six weeks, here in the UK. Otherwise you end up with a secret baby on your hands. Only kidding. I think you just have to pay a little bit more as an admin charge if you're late registering them.

Thanks for playing, quizzer! If you've enjoyed the book, please leave a review on Amazon: it only takes a minute and it really helps (something to do with algorithms, I think)!

Take care and I wish you the very best of luck and happiness in your pregnancy and parenting journey!

- Alex.

OTHER BOOKS BY ALEX MITCHELL

Quizzin' Nine-Nine: A *Brooklyn Nine-Nine* Quiz Book
Parks & Interrogation: A *Parks & Recreation* Quiz Book
Q & AC-12: A *Line of Duty* Quiz Book
Know Your Schitt: A *Schitt's Creek* Quiz Book
Examilton: A *Hamilton* Quiz Book
Stranger Thinks: A *Stranger Things* Quiz Book
The El Clued Brothers: A *Peep Show* Quiz Book
Dunder Quizlin: An *Office US* Quiz Book
A Question of Succession: A *Succession* Quiz Book
The Big Bang Queries: A *Big Bang Theory* Quiz Book
The Greendale Study Guide: A *Community* Quiz Book
Peaky Masterminders: A *Peaky Blinders* Quiz Book

Printed in Great Britain
by Amazon